RECOVERING FROM STROKE

OVERCOMING THE CHALLENGES OF STROKE

DR. MOHAMMAD E. BARBATI

Copyright © 2023 by Dr. Mohammad E. Barbati

All rights reserved.

No part of this book may be reproduced in any form or by any electronic or mechanical means, including information storage and retrieval systems, without written permission from the author, except for the use of brief quotations in a book review.

PART ONE
INTRODUCTION

OVERVIEW: WHAT IS A STROKE?

A stroke is a medical emergency that occurs when the blood supply to the brain is interrupted or reduced, either due to a blockage or rupture of a blood vessel. When this happens, brain cells are deprived of oxygen and begin to die, which can result in significant brain damage and disability.

There are two main types of stroke: ischemic and hemorrhagic. Ischemic strokes occur when a blood clot blocks an artery in the brain, while hemorrhagic strokes result from a ruptured blood vessel in the brain. Ischemic strokes account for approximately 87% of all strokes, while hemorrhagic strokes are less common but often more severe.

The symptoms of a stroke can vary depending on the part of the brain affected and the severity of the stroke. Common symptoms include sudden weakness or numbness on one side of the body, slurred speech or difficulty speaking, confusion or disorientation, difficulty seeing in one or both eyes, and severe headache. It is important to recognize these symptoms and seek emergency medical attention immediately, as the faster a stroke is treated, the better the chances of recovery.

A stroke can have a profound impact on individuals and their families. The physical effects of a stroke can range from mild weakness or numbness to complete paralysis and loss of function. Cognitive effects can include memory loss, difficulty with language and communication, and changes in mood and behavior. These physical and cognitive changes can make it difficult for individuals to perform everyday tasks and lead to a loss of independence.

Stroke can also cause emotional distress, anxiety, and depression for both the individual and their family members. Caregiving for a stroke survivor can be challenging and can lead to increased stress and fatigue. It is important for individuals and families to seek support from healthcare professionals, support groups, and other resources to help them cope with the challenges of stroke.

While stroke can have devastating consequences, it is often preventable. Maintaining a healthy lifestyle, including a balanced diet, regular exercise, and avoiding smoking and excessive alcohol consumption, can significantly reduce the risk of stroke. It is also important to recognize the warning signs of stroke and seek emergency medical attention immediately if symptoms occur. Quick treatment can help reduce the severity of a stroke and improve the chances of recovery.

PREVALENCE OF STROKE AND ITS CONSEQUENCES

Stroke is a leading cause of disability and death worldwide. According to the World Health Organization, there were approximately 13.7 million stroke cases globally in 2016, and stroke accounted for 10.8% of all deaths worldwide. The prevalence of stroke varies by region, with the highest rates in low- and middle-income countries.

In the United States, stroke is the fifth leading cause of death and a leading cause of disability. According to the Centers for Disease Control and Prevention (CDC), there were approximately 795,000 new or recurrent stroke cases in the United States in 2017. This translates to approximately one stroke every 40 seconds.

Certain risk factors can increase an individual's risk of stroke. These include high blood pressure, high cholesterol, smoking, diabetes, obesity, and a family history of stroke. Age, gender, and race are also important risk factors. Individuals over the age of 55, men, and African Americans have a higher risk of stroke.

Stroke can have significant consequences for individuals and their families. The physical effects of stroke can include paralysis, weakness, difficulty speaking, and vision loss. Cognitive effects can include memory loss, difficulty with language and communication, and changes in mood and behavior. These physical and cognitive changes can make it difficult for individuals to perform everyday tasks and lead to a loss of independence.

Stroke can also cause emotional distress, anxiety, and depression for both the individual and their family members. Caregiving for a stroke survivor can be challenging and can lead to increased stress and fatigue.

The economic impact of stroke is significant. In the United States, stroke-related medical costs and lost productivity are estimated to total approximately $34 billion each year. This includes direct medical costs, such as hospitalization and rehabilitation, as well as indirect costs, such as lost wages and productivity.

Preventing stroke is crucial to reducing the burden of stroke. Lifestyle changes, such as maintaining a healthy diet and regular exercise, can significantly reduce the risk of stroke. Managing underlying conditions, such as high blood pressure and diabetes, can also reduce the risk of stroke. Recognizing the signs of stroke and seeking emergency medical attention immediately can improve the chances of recovery and reduce the severity of stroke-related disabilities.

IMPORTANCE OF EARLY RECOGNITION AND TREATMENT OF STROKE

Stroke is a time-sensitive medical emergency, and every minute counts when it comes to treatment. The longer an individual goes without treatment, the more brain cells die, which can result in significant disability or even death. The goal of stroke treatment is to restore blood flow to the brain as quickly as possible to minimize brain damage and improve outcomes.

Recognizing the signs and symptoms of stroke is critical to receiving early treatment. The acronym FAST (Face, Arms, Speech, Time) is commonly used to help individuals recognize the signs of stroke.

There are several treatment options for stroke, depending on the type and severity of the stroke. Ischemic strokes can be treated with medications such as tissue plasminogen activator (tPA) or mechanical thrombectomy, which involves physically removing the blood clot. Hemorrhagic strokes may require surgery to repair the ruptured blood vessel.

The importance of early treatment for stroke cannot be overstated. Time is of the essence, and the sooner an individual receives treatment, the better their chances of recovery. Treatment within the first three hours of symptom onset can significantly improve outcomes and reduce the risk of long-term disability. However, many individuals do not seek medical attention until several hours after symptom onset, which can significantly reduce the effectiveness of treatment.

There are several barriers to receiving early treatment for stroke, including a lack of awareness of the signs and symptoms of stroke, delays in seeking medical attention, and delays in transportation to the hospital. Additionally, some individuals may not receive appropriate treatment due to socioeconomic factors, such as lack of access to healthcare or insurance coverage.

Improving early treatment for stroke requires a multifaceted approach. This includes increasing public awareness of the signs and symptoms of stroke, implementing stroke protocols in healthcare settings to ensure prompt and efficient treatment, and improving transportation and access to healthcare for individuals experiencing stroke symptoms. Telemedicine and mobile stroke units are also emerging as promising strategies to improve early stroke treatment in underserved communities.

PART TWO
UNDERSTANDING STROKE

THE CAUSES, TYPES, AND SYMPTOMS OF STROKE

CAUSES OF STROKE

A stroke occurs when the blood supply to the brain is interrupted or reduced, which can be caused by a blockage or rupture of a blood vessel. The causes of stroke can vary, but some of the most common include high blood pressure, high cholesterol, smoking, diabetes, obesity, and a family history of stroke.

TYPES OF STROKE

There are two main types of stroke: ischemic stroke (embolic or atherosclerosis) and hemorrhagic stroke. Ischemic stroke is the most common type of stroke, accounting for approximately 87% of all stroke cases. It occurs when a blood clot blocks a blood vessel in the brain. Hemorrhagic stroke, on the other hand, occurs when a blood vessel in the brain ruptures and causes bleeding in the brain.

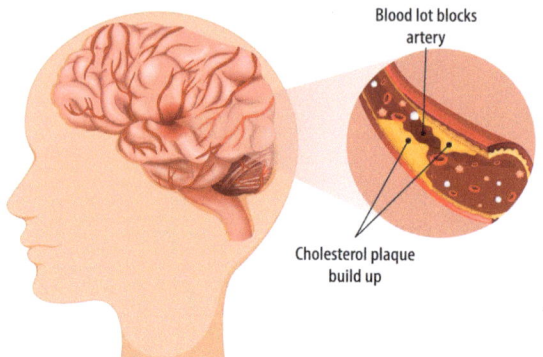

Atherosclerosis Stroke

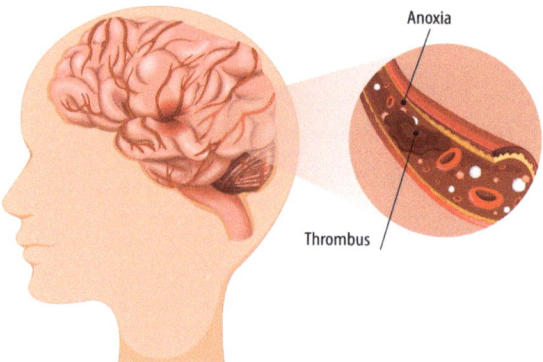

Ischemic Stroke

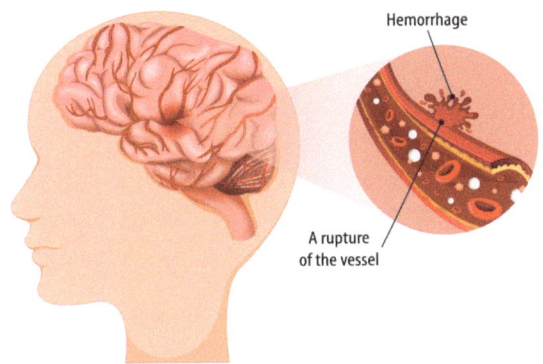

Hemorrhagic Stroke

SYMPTOMS OF STROKE

The symptoms of stroke can vary depending on the part of the brain affected, but there are common signs and symptoms to look out for. These include sudden weakness or numbness in the face, arm, or leg, especially on one side of the body, sudden confusion or trouble speaking, sudden difficulty seeing in one or both eyes, sudden trouble walking, dizziness, or loss of balance, and sudden severe headache with no known cause. Remembering the acronym FAST (Face drooping, Arm weakness, Speech difficulty, Time to call emergency services) can help individuals quickly identify and respond to the signs of stroke.

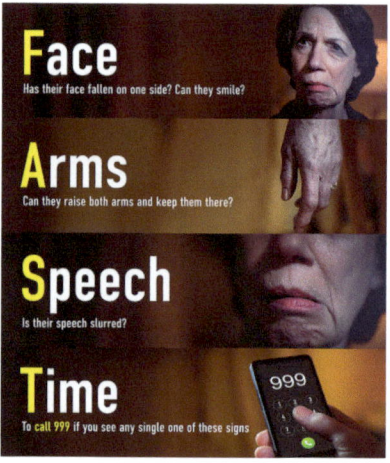

TRANSIENT ISCHEMIC ATTACK (TIA)

A transient ischemic attack (TIA), also known as a "mini-stroke," is a temporary disruption of blood flow to the brain. While the symptoms of a TIA are similar to those of a stroke, they usually last only a few minutes to hours and do not cause permanent brain damage. However, TIA is a warning sign that an individual is at an increased risk of stroke and should seek medical attention immediately.

SILENT STROKE

A silent stroke is a type of stroke that occurs without any noticeable symptoms. While a silent stroke does not cause any immediate symptoms, it can lead to long-term brain damage and increase the risk of future strokes. Individuals who have had a silent stroke may experience changes in cognitive function, such as memory loss and difficulty with language and communication.

Left brain

Right side of body control
- Number skills
- Math/Scientific skills
- Written language
- Spoken language
- Objectivity
- Analytical
- Logic
- Reasoning

Right brain

Left side of body control
- 3D shapes
- Music/Art awareness
- Intuition
- Creativity
- Imagination
- Subjectivity
- Synthesizing
- Emotion
- Face recognition

RISK FACTORS FOR STROKE

Understanding the risk factors for stroke is important for individuals to take steps to prevent the condition from occurring. There are several risk factors for stroke, including lifestyle factors, medical conditions, and genetics.

LIFESTYLE

Unhealthy lifestyle habits can increase an individual's risk of stroke. These factors include smoking, excessive alcohol consumption, lack of physical activity, and an unhealthy diet that is high in saturated and trans fats. Maintaining a healthy lifestyle, including regular exercise and a balanced diet, can help reduce the risk of stroke.

MEDICAL CONDITIONS

Certain medical conditions can also increase an individual's risk of stroke. These conditions include high blood pressure, high cholesterol, diabetes, atrial fibrillation (an irregular heartbeat), and sleep apnea. Individuals with these conditions should work with their healthcare provider to manage their condition and reduce their risk of stroke.

GENETICS

Genetics can also play a role in an individual's risk of stroke. Certain genetic factors can increase an individual's risk of developing conditions that can lead to stroke, such as high blood pressure and high cholesterol. Individuals with a family history of stroke should discuss their risk with their healthcare provider and take steps to manage their risk.

OTHER RISK FACTORS

Other risk factors for stroke include age, gender, race, and previous history of stroke or transient ischemic attack (TIA). Individuals who are older, male, or of certain racial and ethnic backgrounds may be at a higher risk of stroke. Individuals who have previously had a stroke or TIA are also at an increased risk of having another stroke.

DIAGNOSIS OF STROKE

Diagnosis of stroke is crucial for determining the appropriate treatment and developing a recovery plan. Stroke diagnosis involves a combination of medical history, physical examination, and imaging tests.

MEDICAL HISTORY AND PHYSICAL EXAMINATION

Medical history is an important part of stroke diagnosis, as it can provide information about the individual's risk factors and previous medical conditions. During the physical examination, healthcare professionals will assess the individual's neurological function, such as speech, vision, and motor function. They will also check vital signs, such as blood pressure, heart rate, and breathing rate.

IMAGING TESTS

Imaging tests are used to confirm the diagnosis of stroke and determine the type and location of the stroke. The two most common imaging tests for stroke diagnosis are computed tomography (CT) and magnetic resonance imaging (MRI). CT scans can quickly identify whether a stroke is ischemic or hemorrhagic, while MRI can provide more detailed images of the brain.

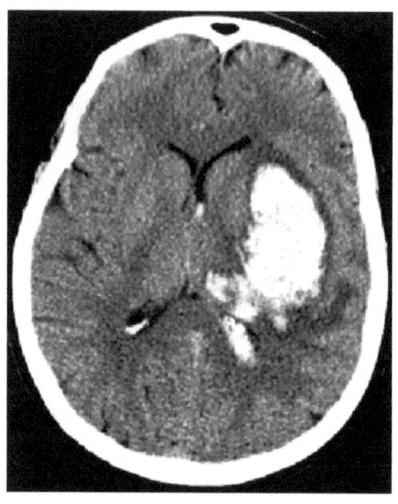

CT scan: Hemorrhagic stroke shown as bright white area

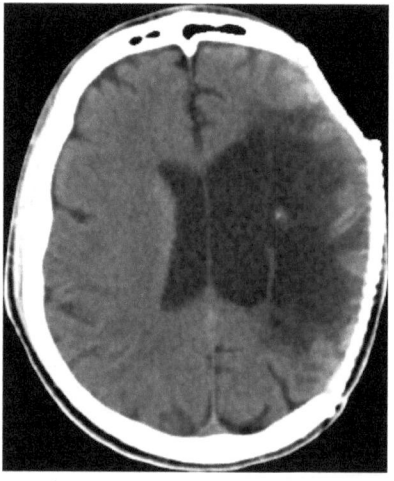

CT scan: An old infarct shown as dark region

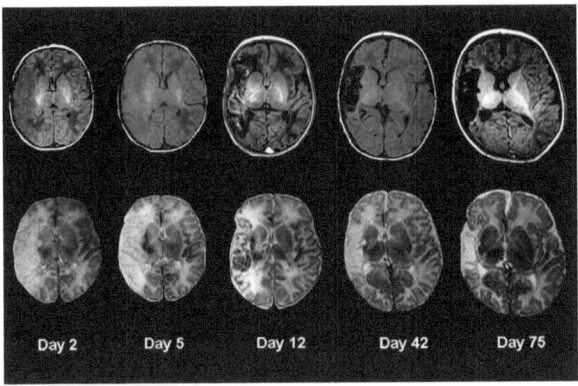

MR scan: Images show the evolution of a right-sided infarction after 2, 5, 12, 42, and 75 days

IMPLICATIONS FOR RECOVERY

Early diagnosis of stroke is crucial for improving recovery outcomes. Treatment for stroke depends on the type and severity of the stroke, and can include medications, surgery, and rehabilitation. Ischemic stroke may be treated with medications that dissolve blood clots, while hemorrhagic stroke may require surgery to stop bleeding in the brain. Rehabilitation after stroke may involve physical, occupational, and speech therapy to improve motor function, daily living skills, and communication.

RECOVERY TIMELINE

The recovery timeline for stroke varies depending on the individual and the type and severity of the stroke. In general, the first few days and weeks after stroke are focused on stabilization and acute treatment. Rehabilitation typically begins once the individual is medically stable and can last for several months or longer. It is important to note that recovery from stroke is often a lifelong process, and individuals may continue to see improvements years after the stroke.

EMOTIONAL IMPACT OF STROKE DIAGNOSIS

Diagnosis of stroke can be a traumatic and emotional experience for both the individual and their family members. Many individuals experience fear, anxiety, and depression following a stroke diagnosis. Healthcare professionals should address the emotional impact of stroke diagnosis and provide resources for coping and support.

PART THREE
THE IMMEDIATE AFTERMATH OF STROKE

THE ACUTE PHASE OF STROKE CARE AND MANAGEMENT

The acute phase of stroke care refers to the first hours and days after a stroke occurs. This phase is critical for preventing further damage to the brain and improving the individual's chances of recovery. Emergency management, assessment, and treatment are key components of acute stroke care, along with monitoring and observation, multidisciplinary care, family education and support, and discharge planning. By providing comprehensive and coordinated care during the acute phase, healthcare professionals can support the individual's recovery and improve their quality of life.

EMERGENCY MANAGEMENT

When a stroke is suspected, it is essential to seek emergency medical attention immediately. Emergency medical personnel will assess the individual's vital signs and provide initial stabilization and support. They will also transport the individual to the hospital for further assessment and treatment.

ASSESSMENT

Upon arrival at the hospital, the individual will undergo a series of assessments to determine the type and severity of the stroke. This will include a medical history, physical examination, and imaging tests such as a CT scan or MRI. The results of these assessments will inform the treatment plan and determine the level of care required.

TREATMENT

Treatment for stroke during the acute phase focuses on restoring blood flow to the brain and preventing further damage. This may include medication to dissolve blood clots or reduce bleeding, blood pressure management, and supportive care such as oxygen therapy or intravenous fluids. In some cases, surgery may be necessary to remove a blood clot or repair a damaged blood vessel.

MONITORING AND OBSERVATION

During the acute phase of stroke care, the individual will be closely monitored for any changes in their condition. This may include frequent neurological assessments, vital sign monitoring, and observation for any signs of complications such as seizures or infections. Intensive care may be required for individuals with severe strokes or who require mechanical ventilation.

MULTIDISCIPLINARY CARE

Stroke care during the acute phase often involves a multidisciplinary team of healthcare professionals, including neurologists, critical care specialists, and rehabilitation specialists. This team works together to provide comprehensive care and support for the individual and their family.

FAMILY EDUCATION AND SUPPORT

The acute phase of stroke care can be a challenging and overwhelming time for individuals and their families. It is important for healthcare professionals to provide education and support to help families understand the diagnosis, treatment plan, and potential outcomes. This may include information about rehabilitation and long-term care options, as well as resources for coping and support.

DISCHARGE PLANNING

As the individual's condition stabilizes, discharge planning becomes an important part of acute stroke care. This may include arranging for rehabilitation services, coordinating with home health services, or providing education and resources for self-care. Discharge planning should involve the individual, their family, and the healthcare team to ensure a smooth transition to the next phase of care.

REHABILITATION DURING HOSPITALIZATION

Rehabilitation plays a vital role in stroke recovery, helping individuals regain their physical, cognitive, and emotional function after a stroke. The rehabilitation team may include a range of healthcare professionals, and rehabilitation strategies may include physical therapy, occupational therapy, speech-language therapy, and psychological therapy. Equipment and technology can also play a role in rehabilitation, and family involvement is important for providing support and assistance. Discharge planning and follow-up care are critical for ensuring ongoing progress and preventing further complications.

GOALS OF REHABILITATION

The primary goal of rehabilitation after a stroke is to help the individual regain as much function and independence as possible. This may include improving physical abilities such as mobility, strength, and coordination, as well as cognitive abilities such as memory, attention, and problem-solving. Rehabilitation also aims to address emotional and psychosocial needs, such as anxiety, depression, and social isolation.

REHABILITATION TEAM

The rehabilitation team typically includes a range of healthcare professionals, such as physical therapists, occupational therapists, speech-language pathologists, psychologists, and social workers. This team works together to develop a comprehensive rehabilitation plan tailored to the individual's specific needs and goals.

REHABILITATION STRATEGIES

There are various rehabilitation strategies that can be used during hospitalization to help individuals recover from a stroke. These may include:

- **Physical Therapy:** Physical therapy focuses on improving mobility, strength, balance, and coordination. Exercises may include range-of-motion exercises, stretching, and strength training.
- **Occupational Therapy:** Occupational therapy focuses on helping individuals regain the ability to perform daily activities such as dressing, bathing, and eating. Activities may include practicing fine motor skills, using adaptive equipment, and modifying the environment to make it easier to perform tasks.
- **Speech-Language Therapy:** Speech-language therapy focuses on improving communication, speech, and swallowing abilities. Activities may include exercises to strengthen the muscles used in speech and swallowing, as well as techniques to improve communication such as using pictures or gestures.
- **Psychological Therapy:** Psychological therapy can help individuals cope with the emotional and psychosocial effects of a stroke, such as anxiety, depression, and social isolation. Therapy may include cognitive-behavioral therapy, supportive therapy, and family therapy.

REHABILITATION EQUIPMENT AND TECHNOLOGY

Rehabilitation may also involve the use of equipment and technology to support recovery. This may include mobility aids such as walkers or wheelchairs, adaptive devices such as eating utensils with larger handles, and technology such as virtual reality therapy or robotics.

FAMILY INVOLVEMENT IN REHABILITATION

Family members can play an essential role in supporting stroke rehabilitation during hospitalization. They can help with exercises, provide emotional support, and assist with activities of daily living. It is also important for healthcare professionals to involve family members in the rehabilitation process, providing education and resources to help them understand the rehabilitation plan and support their loved one's recovery.

DISCHARGE PLANNING AND FOLLOW-UP CARE

Rehabilitation during hospitalization is just the beginning of the recovery process. Discharge planning and follow-up care are crucial for ensuring ongoing progress and preventing further complications. This may involve arranging for outpatient rehabilitation services, coordinating with home health services, or providing education and resources for self-care.

DEALING WITH THE EMOTIONAL AND PSYCHOLOGICAL IMPACT OF STROKE

Stroke not only affects the physical health of an individual but also has a significant impact on their emotional and psychological well-being. It can cause feelings of depression, anxiety, and frustration, not just for the patient but also for their family. Healthcare professionals play a critical role in providing emotional and psychological support to patients and their families, helping them achieve a better quality of life.

EMOTIONAL IMPACT ON THE PATIENT

A stroke can be a traumatic experience for a patient, leading to feelings of sadness, anger, frustration, and even hopelessness. They may struggle to adjust to the changes in their physical abilities, leading to a loss of independence, and a sense of identity. It is crucial for healthcare professionals to recognize the emotional impact of stroke and provide support to the patient.

PSYCHOLOGICAL IMPACT ON THE PATIENT

Stroke can also have a significant impact on a patient's cognitive abilities, leading to difficulties with memory, attention, and problem-solving. These cognitive changes can affect their quality of life and sense of self. Patients may also experience changes in their personality, such as becoming more irritable or impulsive.

EMOTIONAL IMPACT ON THE FAMILY

Stroke not only affects the patient but also has a significant impact on their family members. Family members may feel overwhelmed and unsure about how to provide support to their loved one. They may also experience feelings of guilt, anger, or resentment, leading to strain on the relationship with the patient.

COPING STRATEGIES FOR PATIENTS AND FAMILIES

There are several coping strategies that patients and their families can use to help manage the emotional and psychological impact of stroke. These may include:

- **Seeking Professional Support:** Patients and families can seek support from mental health professionals, such as psychologists or social workers, who can provide therapy and counseling.
- **Joining Support Groups:** Support groups can provide patients and their families with a sense of community and support. They can also offer a safe space to discuss the challenges of stroke and share coping strategies.
- **Encouraging Self-Care:** Patients and their families can engage in self-care activities, such as exercise, relaxation techniques, and mindfulness meditation, to promote emotional and psychological well-being.
- **Maintaining Social Connections:** Patients and their families can maintain social connections with friends and family members to combat social isolation and loneliness.

PART FOUR
LIFE AFTER STROKE

RETURNING HOME AND ADAPTING TO DAILY LIFE

After a stroke, patients often face significant challenges in returning home and adapting to daily life. Returning home and adapting to daily life after stroke can be a significant challenge for patients and their families. However, with the appropriate support and resources, patients can regain their physical abilities, manage their cognitive challenges, and adjust to their new reality. It is essential for healthcare professionals to provide patients and their families with the necessary support and resources to help them achieve a better quality of life.

PHYSICAL CHALLENGES

Patients may experience a wide range of physical challenges following a stroke, including difficulty with movement, balance, and coordination. They may require mobility aids or assistive devices to perform activities of daily living, such as bathing, dressing, and cooking. Physical therapy, occupational therapy, and speech therapy can all play an important role in helping patients regain their physical abilities.

COGNITIVE CHALLENGES

Cognitive challenges, such as memory loss, difficulty with attention and problem-solving, and aphasia, can also be a significant issue for patients following a stroke. Cognitive therapy can help patients improve their cognitive abilities and learn strategies to manage their cognitive challenges.

EMOTIONAL AND PSYCHOLOGICAL CHALLENGES

As we discussed in the previous chapter, stroke can have a significant emotional and psychological impact on patients and their families. Patients may experience depression, anxiety, and frustration, and may struggle to adjust to their new reality. Family members may also experience feelings of guilt, anger, and resentment, and may need support in adjusting to their new role as caregivers.

SUPPORT AND RESOURCES FOR PATIENTS AND FAMILIES

There are many resources available to help patients and their families adjust to life after stroke. These may include:

- **Rehabilitation Services:** Physical therapy, occupational therapy, and speech therapy can all play an important role in helping patients regain their physical abilities.
- **Home Modifications:** Home modifications, such as installing grab bars in the bathroom or widening doorways to accommodate a wheelchair, can make it easier for patients to navigate their home.
- **Assistive Devices:** Assistive devices, such as mobility aids and communication devices, can help patients perform activities of daily living and communicate with others.
- **Support Groups:** Support groups can provide patients and their families with a sense of community and support. They can also offer a safe space to discuss the challenges of stroke and share coping strategies.
- **Mental Health Services:** Patients and families can seek support from mental health professionals, such as

psychologists or social workers, who can provide therapy and counseling.

COPING WITH THE LONG-TERM EFFECTS OF STROKE

Stroke survivors often face long-term physical and cognitive changes that can impact their daily lives. Coping with the long-term effects of stroke can be a significant challenge for stroke survivors and their families. However, with the appropriate support and resources, stroke survivors can manage their physical and cognitive changes and achieve a better quality of life. It is important for healthcare providers to work with stroke survivors and their families to develop a plan for managing the long-term effects of stroke, and to provide ongoing support as needed.

PHYSICAL CHANGES

Physical changes after a stroke can include weakness or paralysis on one side of the body, difficulty with coordination and balance, and fatigue. Stroke survivors may also experience chronic pain or stiffness in the affected limbs. Physical therapy and regular exercise can be beneficial for stroke survivors, as they can help improve strength, flexibility, and balance. Assistive devices, such as walkers or canes, may also be helpful in managing physical changes.

COGNITIVE CHANGES

Cognitive changes after a stroke can include difficulty with memory, attention, and problem-solving. Some stroke survivors may also experience changes in personality or emotional regulation. Cognitive rehabilitation, which involves specific exercises and strategies to improve cognitive function, can be helpful for stroke survivors. It is important for stroke survivors and their caregivers to communicate with healthcare providers about any cognitive changes they experience, as they may indicate a need for further evaluation or treatment.

EMOTIONAL AND PSYCHOLOGICAL CHANGES

Emotional and psychological changes after a stroke can include depression, anxiety, and changes in self-esteem. Stroke survivors may also experience feelings of grief or loss related to the changes in their physical and cognitive abilities. It is important for stroke survivors to seek support from mental health professionals, such as psychologists or social workers, who can provide therapy and counseling. Support groups can also be helpful for stroke survivors and their families, as they can provide a sense of community and support.

LIFESTYLE CHANGES

Following a stroke, stroke survivors may need to make significant lifestyle changes to manage their physical and cognitive changes. This may include changes in diet, exercise, and daily routines. Stroke survivors may also need to modify their home environment to accommodate their physical needs. It is important for stroke survivors and their caregivers to work with healthcare providers and rehabilitation specialists to develop a plan for managing these lifestyle changes.

CAREGIVER SUPPORT

Caregivers play an important role in supporting stroke survivors as they cope with the long-term effects of stroke. Caregivers may experience physical and emotional strain, and may need support in managing their own stress and coping with the changes in their loved one. Support groups and respite care can be helpful for caregivers, as they can provide a break from caregiving responsibilities and a sense of community.

LIFE AFTER STROKE

After a stroke, managing medications, attending follow-up appointments, and making lifestyle changes are essential for reducing the risk of another stroke and achieving a better quality of life. Stroke survivors should work closely with their healthcare providers, rehabilitation specialists, and other resources to develop a comprehensive plan for managing these strategies, and seek support as needed. By taking an active role in their health, stroke survivors can reduce their risk of another stroke and improve their overall well-being.

MEDICATIONS

Medications play a vital role in preventing another stroke. Depending on the type and severity of the stroke, healthcare providers may prescribe medications such as antiplatelet agents, anticoagulants, or cholesterol-lowering medications. Stroke survivors should take their medications exactly as prescribed, and communicate with their healthcare providers about any side effects or concerns. They should also be aware of potential interactions between medications, and inform their healthcare providers of all medications they are taking, including over-the-counter and herbal supplements.

FOLLOW-UP APPOINTMENTS

Follow-up appointments with healthcare providers are important for monitoring stroke survivors' health and managing any underlying medical conditions that increase the risk of another stroke. Stroke survivors should attend all recommended appointments, and communicate any changes in their symptoms or health to their healthcare providers. These appointments may include visits with primary care physicians, neurologists, rehabilitation specialists, and other healthcare providers.

LIFESTYLE CHANGES

Making lifestyle changes can also help reduce the risk of another stroke. This may include adopting a healthy diet, engaging in regular exercise, quitting smoking, and managing other medical conditions such as high blood pressure, diabetes, and atrial fibrillation. Stroke survivors should work with their healthcare providers to develop a plan for making these changes, and seek support from rehabilitation specialists and other resources as needed.

PART FIVE
PREVENTION AND AWARENESS

STRATEGIES FOR PREVENTING STROKE

Preventing stroke requires a combination of healthy lifestyle changes, medications, and surgery in some cases. It's important to work with your healthcare provider to develop a plan that is right for you. By taking steps to prevent stroke, you can protect your brain and body from the devastating effects of this condition.

LIFESTYLE CHANGES

One of the most important strategies for preventing stroke is making healthy lifestyle changes. This includes:

- **Eating a healthy diet:** A diet that is rich in fruits, vegetables, whole grains, lean protein, and healthy fats can help reduce the risk of stroke. Limiting the intake of saturated and trans fats, salt, and added sugars is also important.
- **Exercising regularly:** Physical activity is essential for maintaining good health and reducing the risk of stroke. Aim for at least 30 minutes of moderate-intensity exercise most days of the week.
- **Stopping smoking:** Smoking is a major risk factor for stroke. Quitting smoking is one of the best things you can do for your health.
- **Limiting alcohol intake:** Drinking too much alcohol can increase the risk of stroke. It's important to limit alcohol intake to no more than one drink per day for women and two drinks per day for men.

MEDICATIONS

There are several medications that can help prevent stroke, including:

- **Blood thinners:** These medications help prevent blood clots from forming, which can reduce the risk of stroke.
- **Cholesterol-lowering drugs:** High cholesterol levels can increase the risk of stroke. Cholesterol-lowering drugs can help reduce this risk.
- **Blood pressure medications:** High blood pressure is a major risk factor for stroke. Medications can help lower blood pressure and reduce the risk of stroke.

SURGERY

In some cases, surgery may be recommended to prevent stroke. This includes:

- **Carotid endarterectomy:** This is a surgical procedure that removes plaque from the carotid artery, which can help prevent stroke.
- **Angioplasty and stenting:** This is a minimally invasive procedure that involves placing a small metal mesh tube (stent) in the narrowed artery to improve blood flow and reduce the risk of stroke.

RAISING AWARENESS

Raising awareness about stroke and its warning signs is crucial in the community to ensure that people can recognize the symptoms and seek prompt medical attention. Stroke is a leading cause of death and disability worldwide, and every year, millions of people are affected by it. However, many of these cases could be prevented or treated if people knew the warning signs and acted quickly.

The following are some strategies that can be used to raise awareness about stroke and its warning signs in the community:

EDUCATION CAMPAIGNS

Education campaigns can be an effective way to raise awareness about stroke and its warning signs in the community. These campaigns can include posters, brochures, and other materials that provide information about stroke, its risk factors, and the warning signs to look out for.

COMMUNITY EVENTS

Community events such as health fairs, workshops, and seminars can be used to raise awareness about stroke and promote healthy lifestyle choices that can help prevent stroke. These events can also provide an opportunity to educate people about the warning signs of stroke and the importance of seeking prompt medical attention.

SOCIAL MEDIA

Social media platforms such as Facebook, Twitter, and Instagram can be used to raise awareness about stroke and its warning signs. These platforms can be used to share information about stroke, its risk factors, and the warning signs to look out for. Social media can also be used to share personal stories from stroke survivors, which can help raise awareness about the impact of stroke and the importance of taking preventive measures.

COLLABORATION WITH HEALTHCARE PROVIDERS

Collaboration with healthcare providers can be an effective way to raise awareness about stroke and its warning signs in the community. Healthcare providers can provide information and resources about stroke to their patients and encourage them to take preventive measures. They can also work with community organizations to promote education campaigns and organize community events.

INVOLVEMENT OF COMMUNITY LEADERS

Community leaders such as mayors, city council members, and religious leaders can help raise awareness about stroke and its warning signs in the community. They can use their platforms to promote education campaigns, organize community events, and encourage their constituents to take preventive measures.

AFTERWORD

Overcoming the challenges of stroke is not an easy task, but it is possible. This book has provided valuable insights into the physical, emotional, and psychological challenges that stroke survivors and their families face. It has also provided practical strategies for managing these challenges and achieving a fulfilling life after stroke.

One of the key takeaways from this book is the importance of taking a holistic approach to stroke recovery. This means addressing not only the physical challenges but also the emotional and psychological challenges that can arise after a stroke. It means recognizing that stroke recovery is a journey that requires patience, perseverance, and a support system of healthcare professionals, family, and friends.

Another important takeaway from this book is the power of hope and positivity. Stroke survivors can face many obstacles and setbacks on the road to recovery, but a positive attitude and a sense of hope can help them overcome these challenges. It is important to celebrate the small victories along the way and to focus on the progress that has been made, rather than the setbacks that may occur.

Finally, this book has emphasized the importance of self-care for stroke survivors and their caregivers. Taking care of oneself is essential for maintaining physical and emotional health and for preventing burnout. It is important to prioritize activities that promote well-being, such as exercise, healthy eating, and socializing with friends and loved ones.

In closing, I hope that this book has provided valuable insights and practical strategies for overcoming the challenges of stroke. I encourage you to take a holistic approach to stroke recovery, to maintain a positive attitude, and to prioritize self-care. With these tools and a support system of healthcare professionals, family, and friends, I am confident that you can overcome the challenges of stroke and achieve a fulfilling life after stroke.

ABOUT THE AUTHOR

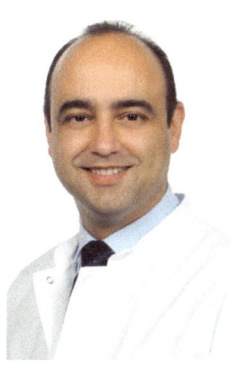

Dr. Mohammad E. Barbati is a consultant vascular and endovascular surgeon. He obtained an MD in endovascular treatment of venous diseases from University Hospital, Aachen. In 2018 he was appointed as a consultant vascular surgeon and lecturer at University Hospital Aachen. Dr. Barbati has been a principal or co-investigator in several clinical trials and studies involving interventional treatment of DVT, PCS, PTS and other vascular diseases. To date, he has authored or co-authored more than 60 scientific publications, abstracts and book chapters. He has given over 100 invited lectures at national and international meetings and is a consultant to many medical device manufacturers.

www.ingramcontent.com/pod-product-compliance
Lightning Source LLC
Chambersburg PA
CBHW040325220526
45473CB00009B/2577